How To Combat Pregnancy Constipation, Morning Sickness & Heartburn

Pregnancy Wellness Handbook: "Managing Constipation, Morning Sickness, and Heartburn with Ease"

By Kimberley Garcia

Copyright

Disclaimer

The material contained in this book is included solely to provide educational and informational content, and it is not meant to serve as medical advice. Readers are strongly encouraged to discuss their health issues and requirements with registered medical experts who are competent in the field.

The author and publisher of this book do not make any claims or guarantees on the correctness, applicability, suitability, or completeness of the information included within this book. For any loss, injury, or damage that may be experienced directly or indirectly as a result of the use or application of any material included in this book, they expressly disclaim any responsibility for such occurrences. Readers are completely accountable for carrying out their acts and making their own choices.

About The Author

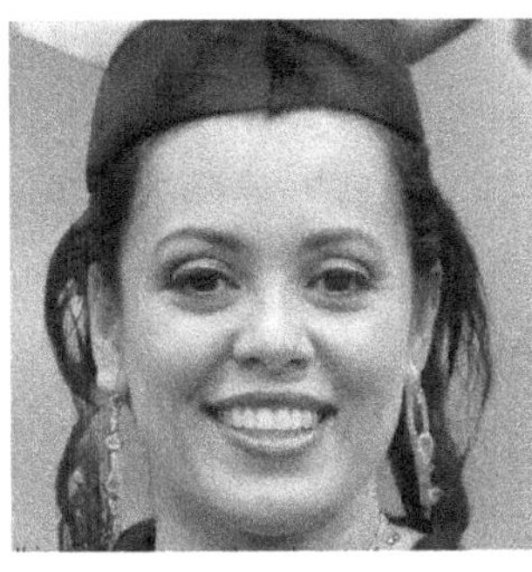

Kimberley Garcia is a devoted medical practitioner who has a strong interest in the health and wellness of women. Throughout the entirety of her professional life, she has been dedicated to delivering compassionate care and encouraging her patients to attain the best possible outcomes for their health. Because Kimberley has a background in obstetrics and gynecology, she has a profound grasp of the one-of-a-kind difficulties and pleasures that come along with being pregnant and a mother.

Kimberley is a committed wife and mother who understands firsthand the joys and complications of managing his job with his family life. In addition to her professional accomplishments, Kimberley is a loving wife and mother. As a result of her personal experiences, she is motivated to share her knowledge and skills with pregnant women to provide support for them during their pregnancy journey.

In her capacity as an author, Kimberley combines her knowledge of medicine with her enthusiasm for writing to produce materials that are both helpful and interesting for women who are expecting. She wants to inspire women to handle the ups and downs of pregnancy with confidence and resilience through the work that she does. She sees her work as a way to demystify pregnancy-related subjects, give practical guidance, and empower women.

When she is not attending to patients or writing, Kimberley takes pleasure in spending quality time with her family, venturing out into the great outdoors, and indulging in her passion for traveling and experiencing new things.

Kimberley's most recent contribution to the subject of women's health is titled "How to Combat Pregnancy Constipation, Morning Sickness, and Heartburn." This book exemplifies her dedication to providing pregnant women all around the world with knowledge and assistance that is supported by evidence.

Table Of Contents

INTRODUCTION

As a pregnant woman, you may experience a variety of discomforts, including constipation, morning sickness, and heartburn. This book is intended to assist you in managing these challenges. Pregnancy is a lovely experience with many changes, but it may also be hard. From dealing with morning sickness to managing constipation and heartburn, the experience of pregnancy can feel like a rollercoaster of physical and mental changes. This guide intends to empower you with the confidence and knowledge to tackle these problems with ease.

As an expecting woman, you may be experiencing new symptoms and may be unclear on how to properly and efficiently alleviate them. This book is here to provide you with practical solutions, professional guidance, and motivating insights to help you handle discomforts connected to pregnancy and embrace the path of parenthood with happiness and strength.

In the next chapters, I will cover the intricacies of morning sickness, including what causes it, what might provoke it, and how to properly live with it. You will learn about several natural therapies, food modifications, and lifestyle adjustments that can help lessen morning sickness and enhance your overall well-being.

Next, we will address the issue of constipation, which is a typical concern for pregnant women. By better understanding the reasons behind constipation and learning practical strategies to aid with regular bowel movements, you will be able to lessen pain and maintain a healthy digestive system during your pregnancy.

Finally, we will discuss the terrible burning sensation of heartburn, which pregnant women regularly suffer. By figuring out what could be causing it, making adjustments to your diet, and discovering safe and effective ways to treat it, you will have the ability to control heartburn symptoms and have a more pleasant pregnancy.

Throughout this book, my purpose is not only to provide you with remedies to common pregnant discomforts but also to give you knowledge, confidence, and a feeling of control over your pregnancy adventure. You will discover practical counsel, recommendations based on science, and helpful assistance to help you tackle the challenges of pregnancy with courage and grace.

This book is a useful guide for pregnant women, whether they are just starting their pregnancy or are nearing giving birth. It includes recommendations on how to deal with typical pregnancy problems, including constipation, morning sickness, and heartburn. By following the suggestions in this book, you can have a healthy and happy pregnancy.

Let's go on this road together and embrace the life-changing experience of being a mother with strength, courage, and joy.

MORNING SICKNESS MADNESS

Understanding Morning Sickness: Causes and Triggers

Morning sickness, typically considered a characteristic symptom of early pregnancy, maybe a trying experience for many pregnant women. Despite its name, morning sickness may occur at any hour of the day, leaving pregnant women feeling nauseated, uncomfortable, and occasionally vomiting. In this chapter, we will study the underlying causes and triggers of morning sickness, shedding light on this prevalent yet puzzling illness.

The Science Behind Morning Sickness

Morning sickness is considered to be predominantly produced by hormonal changes, notably the rise in pregnancy hormones such as estrogen and human chorionic gonadotropin (hCG). These hormonal shifts can impact the gastrointestinal system and the region of the brain responsible for controlling nausea and vomiting, leading to the beginning of morning sickness symptoms.

While the exact processes remain difficult, experts think that hormones play a crucial role in sensitizing the stomach and inducing nausea in reaction to particular stimuli, such as strong scents or specific meals. Additionally, variables including as stress, exhaustion, and variations in blood sugar levels may increase morning sickness symptoms, further confusing the situation.

Recognizing Triggers For Morning Sickness

One of the biggest obstacles in controlling morning sickness is recognizing particular triggers that may increase symptoms. While triggers might differ from person to person, frequent offenders include strong scents, particular meals, and environmental circumstances. Keeping a record of your symptoms and identifying probable triggers might help you determine particular triggers and develop measures to reduce their influence.

Some typical triggers of morning sickness include:

- Strong fragrances, such as cooking smells, perfumes, or cleaning items
- Spicy, oily, or fatty meals

- Foods having strong tastes or textures
- Skipping meals or fasting for lengthy periods
- Stress, worry, or exhaustion

By paying attention to your body's signs and recognizing triggers that increase your morning sickness symptoms, you may make proactive efforts to prevent or reduce exposure to these triggers, therefore minimizing the frequency and intensity of your symptoms.

Coping Strategies For Managing Morning Sickness

While morning sickness can be unpleasant, there are various tactics you can adopt to help control your symptoms and enhance your general well-being throughout pregnancy.

Some helpful coping tactics include:

- Eating small, regular meals to prevent an empty stomach and balance blood sugar levels
- Avoiding factors that worsen nausea, such as strong scents or spicy meals
- Staying hydrated by drinking water, herbal teas, or clear drinks throughout the day
- Getting enough rest and using

> stress-reduction strategies, such as deep breathing or meditation,

- Trying natural treatments such as ginger, peppermint, or acupressure bracelets to ease nausea

By following these coping tactics and making conscious lifestyle choices, you may traverse the challenges of morning sickness with greater ease and comfort, enabling you to focus on the pleasures of pregnancy and prepare for the birth of your little one.

RELIEVING MORNING SICKNESS

The symptoms of morning sickness, which are frequently believed to be one of the most prominent signs of pregnancy, can range from a small feeling of queasyness to a severe feeling of nausea and vomiting. Despite the fact that it is a frequent occurrence and often only lasts for a short period of time, it can have a substantial influence on your quality of life during the first few weeks and months of pregnancy. In this chapter, we will discuss a variety of approaches and treatments that can assist you in overcoming morning sickness and regaining your sense of well-being.

Morning sickness normally starts during the sixth week of pregnancy and tends to reach its height during the first trimester of pregnancy. However, some women may endure morning sickness throughout their whole pregnancy. Hormonal variations, in particular growing levels of human chorionic gonadotropin (hCG) and estrogen, are thought to have a key role in the development of morning sickness, but the precise origin of this condition is yet unknown. A heightened sense of smell, exhaustion, stress, and particular foods or scents can also make symptoms worse. Other variables that might make symptoms worse include fatigue and stress.

Methods Of Coping With Morning Sickness

The management of morning sickness requires a mix of alterations to one's lifestyle, improvements to one's nutrition, and practices of self-care. Some of the simple tactics that can help ease symptoms include eating frequent, short meals to prevent your stomach from being too empty or too full, avoiding triggers such as strong scents or foods that are oily, and getting lots of rest. The process of trying out a variety of meals and beverages to see which ones work best for you, whether it be sour candies, ginger tea, or bland crackers, may also be a source of comfort.

Nutrition Tips To Alleviate Morning Sickness Symptoms

Maintaining good nutrition throughout pregnancy is

vital, especially when suffering from morning sickness. Despite nausea and vomiting, it's crucial to fuel your body with a balanced meal rich in nutrients. Opt for readily digested items that are soothing on the stomach, such as crackers, toast, rice, bananas, and plain yogurt. Sipping on clear fluids like water, herbal teas, or electrolyte-rich drinks might help avoid dehydration, a typical worry during episodes of morning sickness.

Lifestyle Improvements For Minimizing Morning Sickness

In addition to nutritional alterations, several lifestyle improvements can help lessen morning sickness symptoms. Prioritize self-care activities that promote relaxation and stress reduction, such as light exercise, pregnant yoga, meditation, deep breathing exercises, or aromatherapy. Creating a supportive environment that includes understanding family members, friends, or healthcare providers who can give encouragement and aid can also make a huge difference in managing morning sickness.

CONSTIPATION CHALLENGES

Constipation is a frequent and often uncomfortable condition that many pregnant women suffer from. In this chapter, we'll discuss the numerous reasons leading to constipation during pregnancy and present practical solutions for finding relief and supporting gut health.

Understanding Constipation In Pregnancy

During pregnancy, hormonal changes, notably higher amounts of progesterone, might slow down the digestive tract. This slowing gives more time for nutrients to be absorbed, but it can also contribute to constipation as food passes more slowly through the intestines. Additionally, the expanding uterus might impose pressure on the intestines, further leading to constipation.

Dietary Changes To Combat Constipation

One of the most effective strategies to reduce

constipation during pregnancy is to make dietary modifications. Increasing your fiber intake might help add bulk to your stool and support regular bowel motions. Aim to incorporate lots of fiber-rich foods in your diet, such as fruits, vegetables, whole grains, and legumes. Prunes, figs, and bran cereals are particularly beneficial in treating constipation.

Hydration: A Key Factor In Relieving Constipation

Staying hydrated is vital for maintaining healthy digestion and preventing constipation. Adequate fluid consumption helps soften feces, making them easier to pass. Aim to drink lots of water throughout the day, and consider integrating hydrating foods such as soups, broths, and juicy fruits into your diet. Avoid excessive intake of caffeinated beverages, since they might have a dehydrating impact.

Exercise And Movement To Stimulate Bowel Movements

Regular physical exercise is not only excellent for general health during pregnancy but can also help reduce constipation. Gentle workouts, including walking, swimming, and pregnant yoga, help encourage bowel motions and enhance digestive health. Aim for at least 30 minutes of moderate activity most days of the week, with your healthcare provider's consent.

In addition to these lifestyle adjustments, there are also over-the-counter and prescription alternatives available for alleviating constipation during pregnancy. However, it's vital to talk with your healthcare professional before taking any drugs or supplements, as some may not be suitable for use during pregnancy.

By applying these nutritional, lifestyle, and exercise recommendations, you may successfully control constipation throughout pregnancy and ensure optimal digestive health for you and your baby. Remember to listen to your body, remain hydrated, and seek treatment from your healthcare practitioner if constipation continues or becomes severe. With proactive treatment and a comprehensive approach, you may overcome constipation difficulties and have a more enjoyable pregnancy journey.

RELIEVING PREGNANCY CONSTIPATION

Fiber is important for maintaining a healthy digestive system because it helps retain water and aids in moving waste through the intestines. Including fiber-rich foods like cereal, fruits, vegetables, and beans in your diet is beneficial. If you are unable to consume enough fiber through food alone, you can consider taking fiber supplements. Additionally, regular exercise can help improve the movement of your bowels.

If making changes to your lifestyle is not helping with your constipation, you should talk to your doctor about using over-the-counter stool softeners such as Colace. It is important to avoid using laxatives during pregnancy, as they can lead to an imbalance in electrolytes. For hemorrhoids, it is safe to use medicated pads and creams like Tucks and Preparation H.

The Science Behind Constipation In Pregnancy

During pregnancy, hormonal changes, notably an increase in progesterone levels, can slow down the transit of food through your digestive tract. This can contribute to constipation as your body absorbs more water from your diet, making stools firmer and more difficult to clear. Additionally, when your uterus develops, it can put strain on your intestines, further leading to constipation.

Over-The-Counter And Prescription Options For Constipation Relief

If dietary adjustments and lifestyle modifications aren't giving significant relief, your healthcare physician may offer over-the-counter or prescription therapies for constipation. Common alternatives include bulk-forming laxatives, stool softeners, and osmotic laxatives. It's vital to talk with your doctor before taking any medicine during pregnancy to verify that it's healthy for you and your baby.

Herbal Remedies & Supplements For Gentle Relief

Some herbal treatments and supplements may give modest relief from pregnant constipation. Fiber supplements such as psyllium husk or methylcellulose can help boost your fiber consumption, while herbal teas containing substances like senna or dandelion root may induce bowel movements. However, it's vital to be cautious with herbal medicines during pregnancy and contact your healthcare professional before attempting any new supplements.

Lifestyle Modifications To Prevent And Manage Constipation

In addition to dietary changes and exercise, there are numerous lifestyle modifications you may undertake to prevent and manage pregnancy constipation. Establishing a regular toilet pattern, adopting relaxation techniques to reduce stress, and avoiding postponing bowel movements can all help with easier digestion. Experiment with different postures on the toilet, such as raising your feet with a step stool, to maximize bowel motions.

Seeking Medical Assistance For Chronic Constipation Issues

If you have severe or chronic constipation during pregnancy, it's crucial to seek medical assistance soon. Your healthcare professional may analyze your symptoms, rule out any underlying medical concerns, and prescribe suitable treatment choices. In rare circumstances, constipation may be an indication of a more serious disease, such as a bowel blockage or thyroid disorder, needing additional study and therapy.

By using these measures and working together with your healthcare practitioner, you may effectively control pregnant constipation and experience a more pleasant and joyful pregnancy journey. Remember to emphasize self-care, listen to your body, and call out for assistance when required. Your well-being is vital as you start this changing adventure of parenting.

HEARTBURN HASSLES

During pregnancy, heartburn is a typical symptom experienced by many pregnant moms. Characterized by a burning feeling in the chest or throat, heartburn develops when stomach acid backs up into the esophagus. This occurs more frequently during pregnancy because of hormonal changes, increased pressure on the stomach from the developing uterus, and relaxation of the lower esophageal sphincter.

Understanding Heartburn And Acid Reflux During Pregnancy

- Hormonal Changes: During pregnancy, higher amounts of the hormone progesterone can relax the muscles of the digestive tract, especially the lower esophageal sphincter, which ordinarily prevents stomach acid from refluxing into the esophagus.
- Increased Intra-abdominal Pressure: As the uterus grows to support the developing baby, it can put pressure on the stomach, allowing stomach acid to ascend into the esophagus more readily.

- Symptoms of Heartburn: Expectant mothers may suffer a burning sensation in the chest, a sour or acidic taste in the mouth, regurgitation of food or fluids, and discomfort or pain in the upper abdomen or chest.

Identifying Triggers For Pregnancy Heartburn

- Certain meals: Spicy, fatty, or acidic meals can increase heartburn symptoms. Common trigger foods include citrus fruits, tomatoes, chocolate, coffee, and fried or fatty meals.
- Eating Habits: Eating large meals, reclining down quickly after eating, or eating late at night might raise the risk of heartburn. It's crucial to maintain attentive eating habits and avoid overeating.
- Lifestyle Factors: Smoking, heavy alcohol intake, and stress all lead to heartburn symptoms. Making healthy lifestyle choices can help decrease discomfort.

Dietary Modifications To Reduce Heartburn Symptoms

- Eat Smaller, More Frequent Meals: Instead of three large meals, opt for smaller, more frequent meals throughout the day to prevent overloading the stomach and lessen acid reflux.
- Choose Low-Acid Foods: Focus on consuming foods that are low in acidity, such as bananas, apples, oats, whole grains, and lean meats.
- Avoid Trigger Foods: Identify and avoid foods that cause your heartburn symptoms. Keeping a food journal might help you detect particular triggers and make educated dietary decisions.
- Stay Upright After Eating: To lessen the risk of acid reflux, remain upright for at least an hour after eating. Avoid laying down quickly after eating to enable gravity to help keep stomach acid down.

Lifestyle Changes To Minimize Heartburn Discomfort

- Elevate Your Upper Body While Sleeping:

Using extra pillows or a wedge cushion to elevate your upper body while sleeping will help prevent stomach acid from refluxing into the esophagus.

- Wear Loose-Fitting clothes: Tight clothes, especially around the midsection, can put pressure on the stomach and increase heartburn symptoms. Opt for loose-fitting, comfy clothes throughout pregnancy.
- Manage Stress: Stress can increase heartburn symptoms, so it's crucial to use stress-reduction strategies such as deep breathing, meditation, yoga, or light exercise.

By applying these food alterations, lifestyle changes, and coping tactics, you may effectively manage heartburn symptoms and have a more enjoyable pregnancy experience. However, if you encounter severe or chronic heartburn, it's crucial to talk with your healthcare provider to rule out any underlying issues and discuss suitable treatment options.

RELIEVING PREGNANCY HEARTBURN

Heartburn during pregnancy may be a chronic and bothersome condition for many pregnant women. In this chapter, we will study numerous tactics and solutions to reduce heartburn and manage its symptoms efficiently. From over-the-counter pharmaceuticals to natural therapies and lifestyle tweaks, you'll discover a number of solutions to help you get relief and have a more comfortable pregnancy experience.

Over-The-Counter Remedies For Heartburn Relief

1. Antacids: Antacids are routinely used to neutralize stomach acid and give brief relief from heartburn. They are typically regarded as safe during pregnancy when used as indicated. However, it's crucial to pick antacids that are expressly labeled as safe for use during pregnancy and to follow the necessary dose guidelines.

2. H2 Receptor Antagonists: H2 receptor

antagonists, such as ranitidine (Zantac), are another choice for controlling heartburn symptoms. These drugs function by lowering the formation of stomach acid. While they are usually considered safe during pregnancy, it's vital to talk with your healthcare professional before using them, especially if you have any underlying medical issues or concerns.

3. Proton Pump Inhibitors (PPIs): Proton pump inhibitors, such as omeprazole (Prilosec) or pantoprazole (Protonix), may be recommended in situations of severe or chronic heartburn. These drugs act by preventing the formation of stomach acid. While some studies show that PPIs may be used safely during pregnancy, it's vital to assess the possible risks and benefits with your healthcare professional.

Natural Approaches To Alleviating Heartburn Symptoms

1. Dietary Modifications: Certain meals and beverages might increase heartburn symptoms. Avoiding spicy, acidic, or fatty foods, as well as carbonated drinks and

caffeine, may help decrease heartburn flare-ups. Instead, aim for bland, non-acidic meals and beverages that are soft on the stomach.

2. Herbal Remedies: Some herbal medicines, such as ginger or chamomile tea, may give relief from heartburn symptoms. These natural therapies have been used for millennia to ease stomach pain and enhance overall well-being. However, it's crucial to take caution and contact your healthcare practitioner before using any herbal medicines during pregnancy.

3. Lifestyle Modifications: Making minor lifestyle modifications can also help decrease heartburn symptoms. Avoid reclining down quickly after eating, since this might increase the probability of acid reflux. Instead, wait at least two to three hours before lying down or going to bed. Elevating the head of your bed using cushions or a wedge pillow can also help avoid acid reflux during sleep.

Practical Tips For Managing Nighttime Heartburn

1. Sleeping Positions: Experiment with different sleeping positions to find one that reduces heartburn symptoms. Sleeping on your left side may be more pleasant than resting flat on your back or right side, since it can help prevent stomach acid from draining back into the esophagus.
2. Bedtime Routine: Avoid large meals or spicy foods in the hours preceding bedtime. Instead, aim for small, easily digested foods if you're feeling hungry before bed. Additionally, try to relax and unwind before going to sleep, since stress and worry can increase heartburn symptoms.

By adopting these tactics into your everyday routine, you may successfully control pregnancy heartburn and have a more enjoyable pregnancy experience. Remember to contact your healthcare practitioner before making any substantial changes to your food or medication regimen, and don't hesitate to seek medical help if you develop severe or persistent heartburn symptoms. With the correct technique and assistance, you may decrease heartburn discomfort and focus on the joy of pregnancy and impending birth.

CONCLUSION

Congratulations! You've reached the final chapter of "How To Combat Pregnancy Constipation, Morning Sickness & Heartburn." Throughout this book, we've begun on a journey together, exploring the numerous discomforts encountered throughout pregnancy and empowering you with practical techniques to manage them. As you reflect on the amount of knowledge and insights you've gained, let's take a minute to recall important lessons and explore the significance of embracing the journey of pregnancy with enthusiasm and readiness.

Recap Of Key Strategies

1. Understanding Your Body: Pregnancy brings about substantial changes in your body, from hormone oscillations to physical modifications. By obtaining a deeper awareness of these changes and how they lead to discomforts like morning sickness, constipation, and heartburn, you may approach your pregnant experience with greater insight and fortitude.

2. Empowering Self-Care: Self-care is vital throughout pregnancy, both for your physical and emotional well-being. From prioritizing good meals and being hydrated to practicing relaxation methods and seeking assistance from loved ones, self-care plays a critical role in managing pregnancy discomforts and maintaining your overall health.

3. Seeking Support: Remember, you're not alone on this path. Whether you're seeking counsel from healthcare experts, connecting with other pregnant women in support groups, or depending on the support of your spouse and loved ones, reaching out for help may make a huge difference in how you negotiate the obstacles of pregnancy.

4. Flexibility and Adaptability: Every pregnancy journey is unique, and what works for one individual may not work for another. Stay open-minded and be prepared to experiment with different tactics until you find what works best for you. Be kind to

yourself and accept the trip with flexibility and adaptation.

Embracing The Journey

As you prepare to bring your little one into the world, remember that pregnancy is not only about suffering discomforts—it's about embracing the transforming experience of motherhood with grace, strength, and joy. Each milestone, from feeling the first flutter of movement to holding your baby in your arms for the first time, is a monument to the incredible adventure you've begun upon.

Take time to embrace the moments of connection with your developing baby, to cultivate your link with your spouse, and to celebrate the wonder of life emerging inside you. Embrace the changes, both physical and mental, as a monument to the remarkable strength and resilience of the human body.

As you prepare to embark on the next chapter of your journey—parenthood—carry with you the lessons learned, the wisdom gained, and the unflinching belief in your capacity to conquer any difficulty that comes your way. You are capable, you are resilient, and you are deserving of all the love and support the world has to offer.

Thank you for allowing me to be a part of your pregnancy journey. May this book serve as a source of inspiration, wisdom, and support as you navigate the pleasures and trials of pregnancy and embrace the miracle of new life.

I HAVE A REQUEST

Dear **Reader**,

I hope this message finds you well. I am writing to kindly request your feedback and review of my recently published book, **"How To Combat Pregnancy Constipation, Morning Sickness & Heartburn."** Your thoughts and opinions are incredibly important to me, and I would greatly appreciate your honest review.

Your review will not only provide valuable insights but also help other potential readers make informed decisions about whether to explore the book. As a fellow reader, your perspective is highly regarded.

Here's how you can help:

- *Read the Book*: If you haven't already had the chance to read **"How To Combat Pregnancy Constipation, Morning Sickness & Heartburn,"** I'd be happy to provide you with a complimentary copy in your preferred format (eBook or paperback).

- *Share Your Review*: After reading the book, please take a moment to share your thoughts by leaving a review on popular book retail platforms, such as Amazon, Goodreads, or any other platform where you prefer to review books.
- *Be Honest and Constructive*: Your honest opinion is what matters most. Whether you loved the book or had some critical feedback, I welcome your insights. Constructive criticism is just as valuable as praise.
- *Spread the Word*: If you found the book enjoyable and enlightening, consider sharing your review with your friends and family or on your social media platforms to help others discover it.

Your support in providing a review will not only be deeply appreciated, but will also be instrumental in spreading the message and impact of the book. Your input will guide future readers and play a vital role in its success.

Thank you for taking the time to consider my request. Your support means a great deal to me, and I am grateful for your willingness to share your thoughts on **"How To Combat Pregnancy Constipation, Morning Sickness & Heartburn."**

I wish you an enriching reading experience, and I look forward to hearing from you.

Warm regards,

Kimberley Garcia

ADDITIONAL RESOURCES

Dear Reader, I am here again:

Thank you for your support and interest in my book, **"How To Combat Pregnancy Constipation, Morning Sickness & Heartburn."** If you enjoyed this book and are looking for more valuable resources and engaging content, I would recommend some of my books that you might find intriguing:

1. **"Best Parenting Book For Kids With ADHD"**: *An ADHD Parenting Guide for Raising Hyperactive Kids, Dealing with Behavioral Issues, and Supporting Explosive Children*
2. **"Finding Relief"**: *10 Home Remedies To Relieve Menstrual Cramps*
3. **"Successful Parenting Of Kids With Autism"**: *Easy Steps To Raising Brilliant Autistic Kids*
4. **"Single Mom's Pregnancy Guide"**: *A Comprehensive Guide For Single Mothers*
5. **"Pregnancy Cookbook With Nutritional Information"**: *The Complete Healthy Guide*

To Optimal Prenatal Nutrition And Real Food For Pregnancy With 30+ Recipes For Your Pregnancy Meal Plan

6. **"The Complete Guide For Trending Baby Names In 2024"**: *A Thoughtful Up-To-Date Guide To Selecting Unique And Timeless Baby Names For Expecting Mothers, Fathers And Parents*

7. **"Easiest Way To Get Rid Of Pregnancy Hemorrhoids In 2024"**: *Your Essential Handbook For Overcoming Pregnancy Hemorrhoids With Confidence*

8. **"13 Amazing Truths About Pregnancy and Ovulation"**: *Your Roadmap To Successful Conception and Pregnancy*

To explore these books, please visit my Author Central Page on Amazon. **You can scan the QR code below or click the link to visit my Author Central:**

https://www.amazon.com/author/kimberley_garcia

Your continued support means the world to me, and I am committed to providing you with valuable information and inspiration on your journey as a woman.

Thank you for being a part of this community, and I hope my books continue to bring you joy and empowerment.

Warm regards,
Kimberley Garcia

PS: *Don't forget to check out my Author Central page on Amazon to discover more of my books. Your feedback and reviews are always appreciated!*